PRACTICAL TIPS FOR VIBRANT HEALTH:

A Holistic Guide to Nourish Your Body, mind and soul(Optimal wellness)

Gregory Martins

Contents

INTRODUCTION

Welcome to "Practical Tips for Vibrant Health" – your guide to unlocking the transformative power of practical, achievable strategies for a healthier and more vibrant life. In a world filled with information on health and wellness, this b isook stands out as a comprehensive and accessible resource designed to empower you on your journey to optimal well-being.

Embark on a Journey to Wellness:
Are you ready to take charge of your health and embrace a lifestyle that promotes vitality? In these pages, we embark on a journey together, exploring holistic approaches to physical and mental well-being. No matter where you are on your wellness path, whether you're a seasoned health enthusiast or just beginning to prioritize your health, this guide is tailored to meet you where you are.

What Sets This book Apart:

"Practical Tips for Vibrant Health" is not just another health guide; it's a dynamic roadmap crafted to make positive changes accessible and sustainable. Through the lens of practicality, we delve into the intricacies of nourishing your body, incorporating mindful movement, ensuring quality rest, and fostering mental wellness. This eBook is designed to provide you with actionable advice that can seamlessly integrate into your daily routine.

Key Features:

Actionable Insights: Discover practical tips that you can implement immediately, making healthy choices a seamless part of your lifestyle.

Holistic Approach: Embrace a holistic perspective that recognizes the interconnectedness of physical and mental health, offering a well-rounded guide to overall well-being.

Accessible to All: Whether you're a seasoned health enthusiast or a newcomer to wellness, the tips and strategies provided are adaptable to various lifestyles and fitness levels.

Your Wellness Journey Starts Here:

I invite you to dive into the pages of "Practical Tips for Vibrant Health" and embark on a journey that goes beyond quick fixes. Together, let's cultivate a sustainable and vibrant lifestyle that empowers you to thrive physically, mentally, and emotionally. Your path to optimal well-being begins now.

CHAPTER ONE

NOURISHING YOUR BODY

Welcome to the foundational chapter of "Practical Tips for Vibrant Health." In this section, we delve into the essential aspect of nourishing your body, exploring the transformative power of a balanced and nutrient-rich diet. Your journey towards optimal well-being begins with the food choices you make and the nourishment you provide your body.

The Power of Nutrient-Rich Foods:
Fueling your body with the right nutrients is key to vibrant health. In this chapter, we'll explore the importance of incorporating a variety of nutrient-dense foods into your daily diet. From the vibrant colors of fruits and vegetables to the energy-boosting properties of whole grains, we'll uncover the building blocks of a well-balanced and nourishing plate.

Building a Balanced and Sustainable Diet:

Navigating the world of diets and nutrition can be overwhelming. Here, we simplify the process by discussing the principles of a balanced diet. Learn how to create meals that provide the right balance of carbohydrates, proteins, fats, vitamins, and minerals. Discover practical tips for meal planning that suit your lifestyle, making healthy eating both enjoyable and sustainable.

Hydration and Its Impact on Health:
Water is the essence of life, and proper hydration is fundamental to vibrant health. In this section, we'll explore the importance of staying hydrated, not just through water but also through hydrating foods. Learn how adequate hydration supports digestion, skin health, and overall vitality. Practical tips for maintaining hydration throughout the day will be at your fingertips.

What to Expect in This Chapter:

- Insightful discussions on the role of nutrients in supporting various bodily functions.

- Practical tips for incorporating nutrient-dense foods into your daily meals.

- Guidance on building a balanced and sustainable diet that suits your preferences and lifestyle.

- Exploration of the importance of hydration and actionable tips for maintaining optimal fluid balance.

As we embark on this journey to nourish your body, remember that small, intentional changes can lead to significant improvements in your overall health. Get ready to make informed choices that will leave you feeling energized, resilient, and on the path to vibrant well-being. Let's start the transformative process of nourishing your body for a healthier, more vibrant you.

Insightful discussions on the role of nutrients in supporting various bodily functions.

Nutrients are the building blocks of life, playing a crucial role in maintaining the intricate balance and functionality of the human body. In this article, we embark on an exploration of the profound impact that different nutrients have on various bodily functions, shedding light on the intricate web of interactions that contribute to overall health and vitality.

Proteins: The Foundation of Growth and Repair Proteins are the workhorses of the body, serving as the building blocks for tissues, muscles, enzymes, and hormones. This macronutrient is essential for growth, repair, and maintenance of cells. From the muscles that power our movements to the antibodies that defend against infections, proteins are integral to numerous bodily functions.

Carbohydrates: The Energy Source for Daily Activities

Carbohydrates are the primary source of energy for the body. They fuel brain function, support physical activities, and provide the necessary energy for cellular processes. Understanding the role of carbohydrates in maintaining blood sugar levels and the body's glycogen stores is essential for sustaining vitality throughout the day.

Fats: Beyond Energy Storage
Contrary to common misconceptions, fats play a crucial role beyond energy storage. They are essential for absorbing fat-soluble vitamins, supporting brain health, and maintaining the integrity of cell membranes. Different types of fats, such as omega-3 fatty acids, contribute to anti-inflammatory processes and cardiovascular health.

Vitamins: Micronutrients with Macro Impact
Vitamins are micronutrients that act as co-factors in various biochemical reactions. Each vitamin has a specific role, from supporting immune function (Vitamin C) to promoting bone health (Vitamin D) and aiding in blood clotting

(Vitamin K). A well-balanced diet ensures the intake of these essential micronutrients for overall health.

Minerals: The Foundation of Structural Integrity

Minerals are vital for the structural integrity of bones and teeth, nerve transmission, and fluid balance. Key minerals like calcium, potassium, and magnesium are involved in maintaining the body's pH, regulating blood pressure, and supporting muscle function.

Water: The Elixir of Life

Water, while not a nutrient, is fundamental to health. It is involved in nearly every bodily function, from digestion and nutrient transport to temperature regulation and waste elimination. Staying adequately hydrated is paramount for optimal health and vitality.

Conclusion:

In unraveling the intricate role of nutrients in supporting various bodily functions, we gain a deeper appreciation for the importance of a well-balanced diet. The synergy between proteins, carbohydrates, fats, vitamins, minerals, and water is the key to unlocking vitality and maintaining overall health. By making informed and intentional choices in our dietary habits, we empower ourselves to foster a harmonious relationship with the nutrients that fuel our bodies and contribute to a life of sustained well-being.

Practical tips for incorporating nutrient-dense foods into your daily meals.

In the quest for optimal health, the foundation lies in the nourishment we provide our bodies. The choices we make in our daily meals have a profound impact on our overall well-being. In this article, we explore practical tips for incorporating nutrient-dense foods into your daily routine, making healthy eating not just a choice but a sustainable lifestyle.

Start with Whole Foods:

The cornerstone of a nutrient-dense diet is whole foods. Choose unprocessed, minimally refined options such as fruits, vegetables, whole grains, lean proteins, and healthy fats. These foods are rich in vitamins, minerals, fiber, and antioxidants, providing a diverse array of nutrients for optimal health.

Embrace Colorful Variety:
The vibrant colors of fruits and vegetables are indicative of the diverse range of nutrients they contain. Aim to include a variety of colors on your plate, as different hues often signify different types of beneficial compounds. For example, leafy greens are rich in folate, while orange and yellow vegetables often boast high levels of vitamin A.

Prioritize Lean Proteins:
Protein is an essential component of a nutrient-dense diet, supporting muscle health, immune function, and more. Opt for lean protein sources such as poultry, fish, tofu, beans, and

legumes. These options provide a robust nutritional profile without excess saturated fats.

Choose Whole Grains:

Swap refined grains for whole grains to increase the fiber and nutrient content of your meals. Quinoa, brown rice, oats, and whole wheat products are excellent choices that provide sustained energy and essential nutrients like B vitamins and minerals.

Incorporate Healthy Fats:

Not all fats are created equal. Opt for sources of healthy fats like avocados, nuts, seeds, and olive oil. These fats contribute to heart health, aid in nutrient absorption, and provide a feeling of satiety.

Snack Smartly:

Snacking presents an opportunity to add nutrient-dense foods to your daily intake. Choose snacks like Greek yogurt with berries, raw veggies with hummus, or a handful of nuts for a nutritious boost between meals.

Hydrate with Nutrient-Rich Beverages:
Don't forget about what you drink. Water is essential, but herbal teas, infused water with fruits and herbs, and vegetable juices can also contribute to your daily nutrient intake.

Plan and Prep Ahead:
Prepare nutrient-dense ingredients in advance to streamline your meal preparation. Having pre-cut vegetables, cooked grains, and portioned proteins readily available makes it easier to assemble healthy meals throughout the week.

Conclusion:
Incorporating nutrient-dense foods into your daily meals isn't about restrictive diets; it's a celebration of wholesome, delicious, and nourishing choices. By embracing a colorful variety of whole foods, prioritizing lean proteins, and incorporating healthy fats, you're not just nourishing your body – you're cultivating a lifestyle that supports sustained well-being. Start small, experiment with flavors, and enjoy the

journey of nourishing your plate for a healthier, more vibrant you.

Guidance on building a balanced and sustainable diet that suits your preferences and lifestyle.

Embarking on a journey towards a balanced and sustainable diet is a personalized endeavor, uniquely shaped by individual preferences and lifestyles. In this article, we delve into practical guidance on creating a nutrition plan that not only aligns with your preferences but is also sustainable for the long term, fostering a healthier and more vibrant life.

Know Your Nutritional Needs:

Understanding your nutritional needs is the first step towards building a balanced diet. Consider factors such as age, gender, activity level, and any specific health considerations. Consulting with a healthcare professional or a registered dietitian can provide valuable insights into your unique dietary requirements.

Diversify Your Plate:

A balanced diet is built on diversity. Include a variety of food groups to ensure a broad spectrum of essential nutrients. Aim to incorporate fruits, vegetables, lean proteins, whole grains, and healthy fats into your meals. This diversity not only enhances nutritional intake but also adds flavor and excitement to your diet.

Portion Control and Mindful Eating:

Balanced nutrition isn't just about what you eat but also how much. Practice portion control to avoid overeating, and engage in mindful eating by savoring each bite. Pay attention to hunger and fullness cues to develop a healthier relationship with food.

Create a Sustainable Routine:

Sustainability is key to long-term success. Design a dietary routine that accommodates your lifestyle. Consider your daily schedule, work commitments, and social activities when planning meals. Sustainable eating is about finding a rhythm that aligns with your life, making it easier to maintain over the long haul.

Flexibility and Adaptability:
Life is dynamic, and so should be your approach to nutrition. Be flexible in your dietary choices and adaptable to changes in circumstances. Allow yourself the freedom to enjoy occasional treats while maintaining the overall balance in your diet.

Meal Prepping for Success:
Invest time in meal prepping to make balanced choices more accessible. Prepare ingredients in advance, batch-cook meals, and have healthy snacks readily available. This not only saves time during busy periods but also encourages consistency in your dietary choices.

Listen to Your Body:
Your body communicates its needs, and tuning in is crucial for building a sustainable diet. Pay attention to how different foods make you feel.

Notice energy levels, digestion, and overall well-being. Adjust your diet based on these cues to find what works best for you.

Stay Hydrated:

Don't forget the importance of hydration in a balanced diet. Water supports digestion, regulates body temperature, and helps transport nutrients. Aim to drink an adequate amount of water throughout the day, and consider incorporating herbal teas and infused water for variety.

Conclusion:

Building a balanced and sustainable diet that suits your preferences and lifestyle is a dynamic and empowering process. By understanding your nutritional needs, diversifying your plate, and embracing flexibility, you create a foundation for long-term wellness. Remember, it's not about perfection but progress. Find joy in nourishing your body and relish the journey towards a healthier, more balanced you.

Exploration of the importance of hydration and actionable tips for maintaining optimal fluid balance.

Water, the elixir of life, plays a pivotal role in maintaining our health and well-being. In this article, we delve into the significance of hydration and provide practical tips for maintaining optimal fluid balance. From supporting bodily functions to enhancing overall vitality, the journey to hydration harmony is a key aspect of a healthy lifestyle.

Understanding the Importance of Hydration:

Hydration is fundamental to the proper functioning of our bodies. Water is involved in nearly every physiological process, from digestion and nutrient absorption to temperature regulation and waste elimination. Maintaining optimal fluid balance is crucial for overall health, impacting energy levels, cognitive function, and the health of various bodily systems.

The Impact on Physical Performance:

For those engaged in physical activities, staying well-hydrated is particularly vital. Dehydration can lead to fatigue, cramps, and a decline in exercise performance. Whether you're an athlete or someone engaging in regular workouts, maintaining adequate hydration supports endurance, strength, and overall physical resilience.

Cognitive Function and Mood:

Hydration isn't just about quenching thirst; it directly influences cognitive function. Even mild dehydration can impair concentration, alertness, and short-term memory. Sipping water throughout the day can help keep your mind sharp and your mood elevated.

Supporting Digestive Health:

Adequate hydration is essential for proper digestion. Water helps break down food, facilitates nutrient absorption in the digestive tract, and prevents constipation. Maintaining optimal fluid balance supports the digestive system in its intricate processes.

Regulating Body Temperature:

Our bodies regulate temperature through the process of sweating. Staying hydrated ensures an effective cooling mechanism, preventing overheating and contributing to a comfortable and balanced body temperature.

Optimal Fluid Balance for Kidney Health:

The kidneys play a crucial role in filtering waste products from the blood. Hydration supports this process, aiding in the elimination of toxins and preventing the formation of kidney stones. Maintaining an optimal fluid balance is a key component of kidney health.

Actionable Tips for Optimal Fluid Balance:

1. **Listen to Your Thirst Cues:** Pay attention to your body's signals for thirst, and drink water regularly throughout the day.

2. **Carry a Reusable Water Bottle:** Keep a water bottle with you to make hydration convenient, whether you're at work, exercising, or running errands.

3. **Incorporate Hydrating Foods:** Include water-rich foods in your diet, such as fruits (watermelon, cucumber) and vegetables (lettuce, celery).

4. **Set Hydration Goals:** Establish daily hydration goals based on your lifestyle, activity level, and individual needs.

5. **Flavor with Infusions:** Add natural flavors to your water with infusions of fruits, herbs, or a splash of citrus for a refreshing twist.

6. **Monitor Urine Color:** Pay attention to the color of your urine; pale yellow indicates adequate hydration, while dark yellow may signal dehydration.

7. **Hydrate Before, During, and After Exercise:** Prioritize hydration around workout sessions to optimize physical performance and aid in recovery.

Conclusion:

Hydration is a cornerstone of health, influencing various aspects of our physical and mental well-being. By understanding the importance of optimal fluid balance and implementing practical tips, you empower yourself to make hydration a seamless and integral part of your daily life. Strive for hydration harmony and witness the positive impact on your overall vitality and wellness.

CHAPTER TWO

MINDFUL MOVEMENT

In the bustling pace of modern life, the concept of mindfulness has emerged as a powerful antidote to the distractions and stresses that often accompany daily routines. At the intersection of mindfulness and physical activity lies the transformative practice known as mindful movement. This intentional and conscious approach to bodily actions emphasizes a harmonious connection between the mind and body, fostering a heightened awareness of movement, breath, and the present moment. Mindful movement encompasses a diverse array of practices, each offering a unique pathway to cultivating mindfulness through physical engagement. Whether through the flowing postures of yoga, the deliberate sequences of tai chi, or other mindful exercises, the essence remains consistent – to engage in movement with a focused, non-judgmental awareness that transcends the mere physicality of the activity.

This introduction sets the stage for an exploration into the world of mindful movement, where the journey unfolds with deliberate movements, controlled breath, and a commitment to being fully present in each moment. As we delve deeper into the principles and practices of mindful movement, we discover a transformative approach to physical activity that extends far beyond the exercise itself, becoming a holistic pathway to well-being and inner balance.

WHAT IS MINDFUL MOVEMENT?

Mindful movement refers to the intentional practice of physical activities with a heightened awareness of the body, breath, and present moment. It involves consciously paying attention to the sensations, movements, and feelings associated with each action, fostering a deep connection between the mind and body. Mindful movement practices, such as yoga, tai chi, or certain forms of meditation, emphasize a focused and non-judgmental awareness of the body's movements, promoting overall well-being and mental clarity.

Incorporating Exercise into Daily Life

In our fast-paced world, where time is a precious commodity and demands are incessant, finding ways to integrate exercise seamlessly into daily life becomes paramount for our overall well-being. "Move for Life" is an all-encompassing guide designed to empower individuals to effortlessly incorporate exercise into their daily routines. This ebook is a roadmap to cultivating a sustainable and fulfilling relationship with physical activity, making fitness an integral part of your life rather than a chore.

Understanding the Benefits of Daily Exercise

In the modern hustle and bustle of daily life, the importance of regular exercise cannot be overstated. Beyond the obvious physical benefits, daily exercise plays a transformative role in enhancing our overall well-being. This chapter delves into the multifaceted advantages of incorporating exercise into your daily routine, shedding light on its pivotal role in weight management, stress reduction, and improving sleep quality.

Weight Management: Regular physical activity is a cornerstone of effective weight management. Engaging in exercise helps burn calories, contributing to weight loss or weight maintenance. Additionally, it enhances metabolism, making it more efficient in utilizing energy. Strength training, aerobic exercises, and a combination of both have been shown to be effective in managing body weight and composition.

Stress Reduction: In the midst of our fast-paced lives, stress has become a ubiquitous companion. Exercise emerges as a powerful antidote, providing a natural and sustainable means of stress reduction. When we engage in physical activity, the body releases endorphins, often referred to as "feel-good" hormones. These endorphins act as natural stress relievers, promoting a sense of well-being and alleviating tension.

Furthermore, exercise serves as a valuable outlet for accumulated stress and tension. Whether through the rhythmic flow of yoga, the intensity of cardiovascular workouts, or the mindfulness of activities like tai chi, physical activity offers a cathartic release that can significantly reduce the impact of daily stressors.

Improving Sleep Quality: Quality sleep is fundamental to overall health, and exercise plays a crucial role in promoting restful and rejuvenating sleep. Regular physical activity has been linked to improved sleep patterns and a reduction in insomnia symptoms. The relationship between exercise and sleep is bidirectional – not only does exercise enhance sleep, but good sleep also facilitates better physical performance.

Exercise helps regulate circadian rhythms, balances hormones, and reduces symptoms of conditions like sleep apnea and insomnia. However, it's essential to find the right balance, as excessive or vigorous exercise close to bedtime may have the opposite effect. Understanding your body's response to exercise and finding the optimal time for physical activity can contribute to a more restorative and consistent sleep pattern.

OVERCOMING BARRIERS TO EXERCISE
While the benefits of regular exercise are well-established, many individuals encounter barriers that impede their ability to maintain a consistent workout routine. This chapter delves into common barriers to exercise and offers practical solutions to empower individuals to overcome these challenges. By addressing these obstacles head-on, individuals can pave the way for a sustainable and fulfilling relationship with physical activity.

Barrier:

Time Constraints: One of the most common barriers to regular exercise is a perceived lack of time. Busy schedules, work commitments, and family responsibilities often leave individuals feeling overwhelmed and unable to dedicate time to fitness.

Solution:

Prioritize: Recognize the importance of exercise for your overall well-being and prioritize it in your schedule.

Schedule it: Treat exercise as a non-negotiable appointment, scheduling it into your calendar just like any other commitment.

Break it down: If a lengthy workout seems daunting, break it into shorter, more manageable sessions throughout the day.

Barrier:

Lack of motivation: Motivation is a critical factor in maintaining an exercise routine. A lack of motivation can stem from various sources, including boredom, lack of interest, or not seeing immediate results.

Solution:

Set goals: Establish clear, realistic, and achievable fitness goals to provide a sense of purpose and direction.

Find enjoyment: Choose activities you genuinely enjoy to make exercise a more engaging and satisfying experience.

Mix it up: Keep your routine varied and interesting by trying different types of exercises or incorporating new activities regularly.

Barrier:

Overcoming Physical discomfort: Physical discomfort, whether due to existing health conditions, past injuries, or general discomfort during exercise, can deter individuals from engaging in physical activity.

Solution:

Consult a professional: Seek advice from healthcare professionals or fitness experts to create a personalized exercise plan that accommodates any health concerns or limitations.

Choose low-impact options: Opt for low-impact exercises such as swimming, cycling, or yoga, which are gentler on the joints while providing effective workouts.

Barrier:

Lack of social support: The absence of a supportive community or workout buddy can contribute to a sense of isolation and make exercise less enjoyable.

Solution:

Find a workout buddy: Partnering with a friend or family member can make exercise more enjoyable and provide mutual motivation.

Join a fitness class or group: Participate in group fitness classes or sports activities to connect with like-minded individuals and build a supportive community.

Barrier:

Weather and Environmental Constraints: External factors such as adverse weather conditions or lack of access to suitable exercise environments can hinder regular physical activity.

Solution:

Embrace indoor options: Utilize indoor facilities like gyms, fitness studios, or home workouts during inclement weather.

Equip yourself for outdoor exercise: Invest in weather-appropriate gear to make outdoor activities more comfortable, regardless of the conditions.

FINDING YOUR FITNESS PASSION

Embarking on a journey toward a healthier lifestyle involves discovering physical activities that resonate with your interests and preferences. This chapter explores the importance of finding your fitness passion and provides guidance on uncovering enjoyable and sustainable forms of exercise. By aligning your workouts with activities that bring you joy, you enhance your motivation and make exercise an integral and fulfilling part of your life.

1. Understanding the Significance of Passion:
Understanding the significance of finding your fitness passion goes beyond simply engaging in physical activity. It taps into the emotional and psychological aspects of exercise, transforming it from a routine obligation into a source of genuine enjoyment. When you discover activities that resonate with your interests, you are more likely to stay committed and make exercise a lifelong pursuit.

2. Exploring Various Exercise Modalities:

To find your fitness passion, it's essential to explore a variety of exercise modalities. The world of fitness is diverse, offering an array of activities to suit different preferences and fitness levels. Some popular options include:

- Cardiovascular activities: Running, cycling, dancing, or group fitness classes.

- Strength training: Weightlifting, resistance training, or bodyweight exercises.

- Mind-body exercises: Yoga, Pilates, or tai chi.

- Outdoor activities: Hiking, swimming, or team sports.

3. Assessing Personal Interests and Preferences:

To discover your fitness passion, consider your personal interests and preferences. Reflect on activities you enjoyed in the past, hobbies you are drawn to, and the environments where you feel most comfortable. This self-assessment will guide you toward activities that align with your individual tastes and make exercise an enjoyable and sustainable part of your routine.

4. Trying New Activities:

Finding your fitness passion may involve trying new activities that you haven't considered before. Be open to experimentation and embrace a mindset of exploration. Attend different fitness classes, join sports clubs, or experiment with home workout routines to broaden your horizons and uncover activities that resonate with you.

5. Paying Attention to Enjoyment:

The key indicator of your fitness passion is the level of enjoyment you experience during and after an activity. Pay attention to how you feel both physically and mentally. If an activity brings you joy, boosts your mood, and leaves you looking forward to the next session, you're on the right trtrack.

6. **Personalizing Your Fitness Journey:**
The journey to finding your fitness passion is a deeply personal one. It's not about adhering to societal expectations or trends but about discovering what genuinely fulfills you. Personalize your fitness journey by incorporating elements that bring you joy, whether it's dancing to your favorite music, practicing mindfulness through yoga, or challenging yourself with strength training.

MAKING EXERCISE A DAILY HABIT

The transition from sporadic workouts to making exercise a daily habit is a pivotal step in cultivating a healthy and active lifestyle. This chapter delves into the significance of turning exercise into a routine and provides practical tips for establishing a consistent workout regimen. By transforming physical activity into a daily habit, individuals can harness the power of routine to enhance overall well-being and make exercise an integral part of their daily lives.

i) Understanding the Power of Habits:
Habits are powerful drivers of behavior, offering a framework that requires less conscious effort over time. Turning exercise into a daily habit leverages the inherent consistency and predictability of routines, making it easier to prioritize physical activity amidst the demands of daily life.

ii) Setting Realistic and Achievable Goals:
The foundation of a daily exercise habit begins with setting realistic and achievable goals. Break down your fitness aspirations into smaller, manageable milestones. Whether it's increasing daily steps, committing to a 20-minute workout, or incorporating regular stretching, establishing achievable goals sets the stage for habit formation.

iii) Identifying a Consistent Time:
Consistency is key to habit formation, and identifying a consistent time for exercise helps integrate it seamlessly into your daily routine.

Whether it's early morning, during lunch, or in the evening, choose a time that aligns with your schedule and energy levels. Consistency fosters routine, making exercise a non-negotiable part of your day.

iv) Preparing in Advance:
Minimize obstacles by preparing for your exercise routine in advance. Lay out workout clothes the night before, pack a gym bag, or have home workout equipment readily accessible. Removing logistical barriers makes it easier to transition seamlessly from daily activities to exercise.

V) Starting Small and Gradually Progressing:
Begin your journey toward a daily exercise habit by starting small. Rather than overwhelming yourself with intense workouts, initiate the habit with manageable activities. As your routine becomes ingrained, gradually increase the intensity, duration, or frequency of your workouts. Small, consistent steps lead to sustainable progress.

Vi) Incorporating Enjoyable Activities:
Make exercise a daily habit by incorporating activities you genuinely enjoy. When you look forward to your workouts, they become more than a task; they become a source of pleasure. Whether it's dancing, hiking, or participating in group classes, finding joy in your chosen activities enhances the likelihood of forming a lasting habit.

Vii) Accountability and Support:
Enlist the support of friends, family, or workout buddies to enhance accountability. Share your goals and progress with others who can provide encouragement and motivation. Group activities, fitness classes, or virtual challenges are effective ways to create a supportive community around your exercise routine.

Viii) Tracking Progress:
Track your progress to celebrate achievements and reinforce the habit. Whether through a fitness app, journal, or wearable device,

monitoring your workouts provides a visual representation of your commitment and accomplishments, motivating you to continue the habit.

SNEAKING IN EXERCISE THROUGHOUT THE DAY

In the midst of busy schedules and sedentary lifestyles, the concept of sneaking in exercise throughout the day offers a practical and creative solution to enhance physical activity. This chapter explores the importance of infusing movement into everyday tasks and provides creative ways to seamlessly integrate exercise into various facets of daily life. By adopting a holistic approach to physical activity, individuals can accumulate moments of exercise that collectively contribute to a healthier and more active lifestyle.

The Importance of Continuous Movement:

Sneaking in exercise throughout the day is rooted in the understanding that consistent movement is beneficial for overall health. Instead of relying solely on dedicated workout sessions, incorporating physical activity into daily tasks maintains a steady level of movement, promoting better circulation, improved energy levels, and enhanced overall well-being.

For those with sedentary jobs, incorporating desk exercises and active breaks can be transformative. Simple stretches, leg lifts, or seated exercises can be discreetly integrated into your workday, preventing prolonged periods of inactivity and promoting circulation. Set reminders to take short breaks to stand, stretch, or walk around every hour.

Active Commuting:
Transforming your daily commute into an active endeavor is an effective way to sneak in exercise. Consider walking or cycling to work, using public transportation with additional

walking involved, or parking farther away from your destination. These subtle changes accumulate significant physical activity over time.

Stair Climbing:

Take advantage of staircases as an opportunity for exercise. Opt for stairs instead of elevators whenever possible, or deliberately add a few flights of stairs to your daily routine. Stair climbing engages multiple muscle groups and provides a cardiovascular boost without the need for dedicated workout time.

Household Chores as Workouts:

Household chores offer a dual benefit by contributing to a tidy living space and serving as opportunities for physical activity. Engage in activities like vacuuming, sweeping, or gardening, which involve bending, lifting, and moving, effectively turning chores into mini-workouts.

Fitness Microbursts:

Incorporate fitness microbursts into your day by performing quick, high-intensity exercises. These can include short bouts of jumping jacks, squats, or lunges. Schedule these microbursts strategically throughout the day to elevate your heart rate and invigorate your body.

Incorporating Playful Movement:
Rediscover the joy of playful movement by engaging in activities like dancing, playing with pets, or joining children in active play. Playful movements not only contribute to physical activity but also infuse moments of joy and spontaneity into your day.

Utilizing Technology for Reminders:
Leverage technology to set reminders for brief exercise breaks. Apps, smartwatches, or simple phone alarms can prompt you to stand up, stretch, or perform quick exercises, reinforcing the habit of sneaking in physical activity.

CREATING A SUPPORTING ENVIRONMENT

In the pursuit of a regular exercise routine, the environment in which you live, work, and socialize plays a pivotal role. This chapter explores the importance of a supportive environment in fostering a culture of regular exercise and provides strategies for creating surroundings that encourage and sustain physical activity. A supportive environment can be a powerful catalyst for making exercise an integral part of daily life, promoting consistency, motivation, and overall well-being.

The Influence of Environment on Behavior: Research consistently highlights the profound impact that environment has on individual behaviors. When the spaces we inhabit are conducive to physical activity, the likelihood of engaging in regular exercise significantly increases. Conversely, environments that discourage movement may pose barriers to the establishment of a consistent workout routine.

Home Environment:

Your home environment serves as the primary backdrop for daily activities. Transform it into a supportive space for exercise by:

- **Designating a workout area:** Dedicate a specific area in your home for exercise, whether it's a corner with a yoga mat or a room with workout equipment.
- **Investing in home workout tools:** Equip your home with basic exercise tools like resistance bands, dumbbells, or a stability ball.
- **Displaying visual cues:** Place motivational quotes, fitness goals, or a workout schedule in visible locations to inspire and remind you of your commitment to exercise.

Workplace Environment:

The workplace is another influential setting that can either facilitate or hinder regular exercise. Foster a supportive workplace environment by:

- **Encouraging active breaks:** Advocate for short breaks during the workday for stretching, walking, or quick exercises to combat sedentary habits.
- **Utilizing ergonomic tools:** Invest in ergonomic office furniture and tools that promote movement, such as standing desks or stability ball chairs.

Social Environment:

The influence of social connections on behavior is profound. Leverage your social environment for support:

- **Forming exercise groups:** Join or create exercise groups with friends, family, or colleagues to foster a sense of community and accountability.
- **Participating in fitness classes or clubs:** Engage in group fitness classes or join local clubs that align with your interests, making exercise a social and enjoyable activity.

Community Environment:

The broader community in which you live contributes to the opportunities and resources available for physical activity:

- **Exploring local parks and trails:** Take advantage of nearby parks and trails for outdoor activities like walking, jogging, or cycling.
- **Accessing fitness facilities:** Consider proximity to gyms, fitness studios, or recreational facilities when choosing your residence.

Virtual Support:
In the digital age, virtual environments also play a role in shaping our behaviors:
- **Joining online fitness communities:** Participate in virtual fitness communities or social media groups that provide support, inspiration, and shared experiences.
- **Using fitness apps:** Utilize fitness apps that offer workout routines, progress

tracking, and reminders, enhancing the virtual support for your exercise journey.

Establishing Supportive Rituals:

Create daily or weekly rituals that support your exercise routine:

- **Scheduling regular workout times:** Consistently schedule exercise sessions to establish a routine that becomes ingrained in your daily or weekly schedule.
- **Incorporating family or friends:** Involve family or friends in your exercise rituals, making physical activity a shared experience.

TAILORING EXERCISE TO YOUR LIFESTYLE

Achieving and maintaining a regular exercise routine hinges on the ability to tailor physical activity to your unique lifestyle. This chapter delves into the importance of aligning exercise with your individual schedule, preferences, and daily demands. By developing a personalized exercise plan that integrates seamlessly into your lifestyle, you not only enhance the likelihood of consistency but also foster a sustainable and enjoyable approach to fitness.

Recognizing Individual Lifestyle Factors:
Every individual possesses a distinct lifestyle characterized by varied schedules, responsibilities, and preferences. Recognizing these unique factors is the first step in tailoring exercise to your lifestyle. Consider aspects such as:

- Work schedule
- Family commitments
- Personal interests
- Time of day preferences
- Existing hobbies and activities

Assessing Time Constraints:
Time is often a significant factor influencing exercise adherence. Assess your daily and weekly schedule to identify pockets of time available for physical activity. Recognize that

effective workouts need not be lengthy; even short, focused sessions can yield substantial benefits.

Identifying Preferred Exercise Modalities:
Tailoring exercise to your lifestyle involves selecting activities that align with your preferences and interests. Explore various exercise modalities, such as:

- Cardiovascular exercises: Running, cycling, dancing
- Strength training: Weightlifting, bodyweight exercises
- Mind-body exercises: Yoga, Pilates, tai chi
- Outdoor activities: Hiking, swimming, team sports

Choosing activities you enjoy enhances the likelihood of making exercise a consistent and fulfilling part of your routine.

Integrating Exercise into Daily Rituals:

Incorporate exercise seamlessly into existing daily rituals to overcome time constraints. Strategies include:

- Morning routines: Perform a quick workout, stretch, or yoga session upon waking.
- Lunch breaks: Utilize breaks for a brisk walk or quick bodyweight exercises.
- Evening wind-down: Engage in calming activities like yoga or gentle stretching before bedtime.

Prioritizing Consistency Over Intensity:
Tailoring exercise to your lifestyle involves prioritizing consistency over intensity. Instead of focusing solely on vigorous workouts, strive for regular, moderate exercise that aligns with your energy levels and daily commitments. Consistency builds habits, fostering a sustainable approach to fitness.

Incorporating Functional Exercises:

Functional exercises mimic daily movements, making them highly relevant to your lifestyle. These exercises enhance overall functionality and can be seamlessly integrated into your routine. Examples include squats, lunges, and core-strengthening exercises.

Setting Realistic Goals:

Developing a personalized exercise plan requires setting realistic and achievable goals. Align your fitness aspirations with your lifestyle, considering factors like:

- Frequency of workouts per week
- Duration of each session
- Desired outcomes (weight loss, strength building, flexibility)
- Realistic goals contribute to a sense of accomplishment and motivation.

Adapting to Changes:

Life is dynamic, and your exercise plan should be adaptable. Be open to adjusting your routine based on changes in work, family, or personal circumstances. Flexibility ensures that your exercise plan remains feasible and enjoyable in the long run.

CHAPTER THREE

REST AND RECOVERY

In the exhilarating pursuit of personal and professional goals, the concept of rest and recovery often takes a backseat to the prevailing ethos of productivity and achievement. However, in the intricate tapestry of a well-balanced and fulfilling life, the importance of intentional rest and thoughtful recovery cannot be overstated. This introductory exploration delves into the transformative power of embracing rest as not just a momentary pause but as a deliberate and essential component of holistic well-being.

The Misconception of Constant Motion

In a world that celebrates constant motion and perpetual progress, the idea of slowing down, pausing, and rejuvenating may appear counterintuitive. Yet, athletes, scholars, and individuals at the pinnacle of their fields understand that peak performance is intricately woven with adequate periods of rest and recovery. Contrary to popular belief, rest is not synonymous with idleness; it is a strategic, purposeful act that propels us forward with renewed vigor.

The Physical and Mental Rebirth

Rest and recovery extend far beyond the realm of physical rejuvenation. While they play a crucial role in healing muscles and preventing burnout, their impact transcends the physical domain. Adequate rest is the crucible in which creativity is sparked, resilience is forged, and mental acuity is sharpened. It is the secret ingredient that nurtures emotional well-being and fosters the fortitude needed to navigate life's challenges.

In this chapters, we will delve into the importance of quality sleep, stress management techniques, and creating a relaxing bedtime routine.

Importance Of Quality Sleep

In the frenetic pace of modern life, where productivity and achievement often take center stage, one fundamental aspect of well-being tends to be overshadowed – the quality of our sleep. Sleep is not merely a passive state of rest; it is a dynamic and intricate process that plays a vital role in supporting physical health, cognitive function, emotional balance, and overall longevity. In this exploration, we delve into the profound importance of quality sleep and its far-reaching impact on every facet of our lives.

The Science of Sleep:

Quality sleep is a complex interplay of physiological and neurological processes that occur during different sleep stages. It involves cycles of rapid eye movement (REM) and non-REM sleep, each contributing to essential functions such as memory consolidation, hormone regulation, and cellular repair. The intricate dance of neurotransmitters and hormones orchestrates a symphony of restoration while we slumber.

Cognitive Function and Memory:

One of the most tangible benefits of quality sleep is its transformative effect on cognitive function and memory. During REM sleep, the brain consolidates and stores information acquired throughout the day, facilitating learning and knowledge retention. Lack of adequate sleep, on the other hand, impairs these processes, leading to diminished concentration, memory lapses, and decreased cognitive performance.

Physical Restoration and Immune Function:

Beyond cognitive benefits, quality sleep is paramount for physical restoration and immune function. During deep sleep, the body undergoes repair and regeneration, including the release of growth hormone essential for tissue repair, muscle growth, and overall maintenance. Adequate sleep also supports a robust immune system, enhancing the body's ability to fend off infections and diseases.

Emotional Well-Being and Mental Health:

Sleep and mental health share a bidirectional relationship. Quality sleep fosters emotional resilience, while the lack thereof can contribute to mood disturbances, heightened stress levels, and an increased risk of mental health disorders. Chronic sleep deprivation has been linked to conditions such as anxiety, depression, and an elevated risk of developing mood disorders.

Hormonal Balance and Weight Management:
Sleep plays a crucial role in regulating hormones that influence appetite and metabolism. Disruptions in sleep patterns can lead to imbalances in ghrelin and leptin, the hormones responsible for hunger and satiety. Consequently, sleep deprivation may contribute to weight gain, obesity, and an increased risk of metabolic disorders.

The Importance of Sleep Hygiene:
Quality sleep is not solely about quantity; it also hinges on the practice of good sleep hygiene. This involves cultivating habits and creating an environment conducive to restful sleep. Key

elements of sleep hygiene include maintaining a consistent sleep schedule, creating a comfortable sleep environment, limiting exposure to electronic devices before bedtime, and avoiding stimulants like caffeine close to sleep.

Embracing the Art of Prioritizing Sleep:
In a culture that often celebrates burning the midnight oil, the art of prioritizing sleep emerges as a counterintuitive yet indispensable practice. Recognizing the importance of quality sleep is an empowering decision to invest in our physical and mental well-being. It involves carving out dedicated time for sleep, establishing a calming bedtime routine, and fostering an environment that promotes rest.

Conclusion:

The Gateway to Holistic Well-Being
Quality sleep is the unsung hero of holistic well-being, influencing every aspect of our lives. As we unravel the profound importance of sleep, we unveil a gateway to enhanced cognitive function, emotional resilience, physical vitality,

and mental health. Embracing the art of prioritizing sleep is not a luxury; it is a foundational investment in our present and future selves. In the subsequent chapters, we will delve into practical strategies for improving sleep quality, exploring mindfulness techniques, and cultivating habits that honor the transformative power of a good night's rest.

Stress Management

In the dynamic tapestry of modern life, stress has become an ever-present companion, impacting our mental, emotional, and physical well-being. The ability to navigate stress is a crucial skill, and fortunately, there exists a rich repertoire of stress management techniques that empower individuals to restore balance, cultivate resilience, and foster a sense of tranquility. This article explores a diverse array of effective stress management techniques, offering a roadmap to navigate the complexities of daily life with poise and grace.

Understanding Stress:

Before delving into stress management techniques, it's essential to grasp the nature of stress. Stress, in its essence, is the body's natural response to challenges and demands. While acute stress can be a motivator and enhancer of performance, chronic stress can lead to a cascade of detrimental effects on physical and mental health. Effectively managing stress involves adopting strategies that address its root causes while enhancing one's capacity to cope.

Mindfulness and Meditation:

At the forefront of stress management techniques lies mindfulness and meditation. These practices, rooted in ancient traditions, involve cultivating a heightened awareness of the present moment. Mindfulness encourages non-judgmental observation of thoughts and feelings, fostering a sense of calm amidst life's tumult. Meditation, whether through focused breathwork, guided imagery, or mantra repetition, provides a sanctuary for the mind, allowing it to unwind and recalibrate.

Progressive Muscle Relaxation (PMR):
Progressive Muscle Relaxation is a systematic technique that involves tensing and then relaxing different muscle groups, promoting physical relaxation and alleviating tension. By progressively releasing muscle tension throughout the body, PMR induces a corresponding sense of calm in the mind, making it a valuable tool for stress relief.

Deep Breathing Exercises:
Conscious control of the breath is a powerful stress management technique. Deep breathing exercises, such as diaphragmatic breathing or the 4-7-8 technique, engage the body's parasympathetic nervous system, eliciting a relaxation response. Regular practice of deep breathing can mitigate the physiological effects of stress and enhance overall well-being.

Physical Exercise:

Physical activity is a potent antidote to stress, as it releases endorphins, the body's natural mood enhancers. Engaging in regular exercise, whether through aerobic activities like running or cycling or more meditative practices like yoga, not only reduces stress levels but also contributes to improved overall mental health.

Time Management and Prioritization:

A significant source of stress often stems from feeling overwhelmed by an abundance of tasks and responsibilities. Effective time management and prioritization techniques, such as creating to-do lists, breaking tasks into manageable steps, and setting realistic goals, empower individuals to regain a sense of control over their schedules, reducing stress in the process.

Social Connection and Support:

Human connection serves as a crucial buffer against stress. Cultivating and nurturing relationships with friends, family, or support groups provides an emotional safety net during challenging times. Sharing concerns, seeking advice, or simply enjoying companionship can significantly alleviate stress and foster a sense of belonging.

Cognitive Behavioral Techniques (CBT):
Cognitive Behavioral Therapy is a therapeutic approach that helps individuals identify and change negative thought patterns and behaviors contributing to stress. By challenging and reframing irrational beliefs, CBT empowers individuals to develop healthier coping mechanisms and responses to stressors.

Art and Creativity:
Engaging in artistic and creative pursuits offers a unique avenue for stress relief. Whether through painting, writing, music, or other forms of self-expression, the creative process provides an outlet for emotions, allowing individuals to channel stress into a positive and fulfilling endeavor.

Nature and Outdoor Activities:

Reconnecting with nature and engaging in outdoor activities has a profound impact on stress reduction. Spending time in natural settings, whether it's a walk in the park or a weekend hike, has been shown to lower cortisol levels and promote a sense of tranquility.

Seeking Professional Support:
In cases of persistent or overwhelming stress, seeking professional support is a courageous and essential step. Mental health professionals, including therapists, counselors, and psychologists, can provide tailored strategies and interventions to address specific stressors and build resilience.

Conclusion: Weaving a Tapestry of Resilience
Effectively managing stress is a dynamic and individualized process. By incorporating a combination of these stress management techniques into one's daily routine, individuals can weave a tapestry of resilience that empowers them to navigate life's challenges with grace and equanimity. As we embrace these techniques, we

embark on a journey towards greater well-being, fostering not only the ability to manage stress but also to cultivate a profound sense of inner peace.

Creating A Relaxing Bedtime Routine

In the hustle and bustle of daily life, the transition from the demands of the day to a peaceful night's sleep often requires intentional and calming rituals. A relaxing bedtime routine serves as a bridge between the busyness of the outside world and the serenity of the night, allowing us to unwind, release the tensions of the day, and prepare our minds and bodies for restorative sleep. This article explores the art of crafting a tranquil evening routine that promotes relaxation and sets the stage for a restful night.

1. Establish a Consistent Sleep Schedule:

The foundation of a relaxing bedtime routine begins with consistency. Set a regular sleep schedule by going to bed and waking up at the same time every day, even on weekends. This helps regulate your body's internal clock, optimizing the quality of your sleep.

2. Create a Comfortable Sleep Environment:
Transform your bedroom into a sanctuary of tranquility. Invest in a comfortable mattress and pillows, choose soft bedding, and adjust the room temperature to your preference. Dim the lights in the evening to signal to your body that it's time to wind down.

3. Unplug from Electronic Devices:
The blue light emitted by electronic devices can interfere with the production of the sleep-inducing hormone melatonin. Establish a technology curfew an hour before bedtime, allowing your mind to detach from the digital world and facilitating a smoother transition into sleep.

4. Gentle Pre-Sleep Activities:

Engage in calming activities that signal the winding down of the day. Reading a book, practicing gentle stretching or yoga, or listening to soothing music are excellent pre-sleep rituals. Choose activities that help quiet the mind and relax the body.

5. Mindful Breathing and Meditation:
Incorporate mindfulness techniques into your bedtime routine to cultivate a sense of calm. Mindful breathing exercises or a short meditation can help center your thoughts and release any lingering tension from the day, promoting a tranquil state of mind.

6. A Warm Bath or Shower:
A warm bath or shower before bedtime can be a luxurious and effective way to relax your muscles and signal to your body that it's time for sleep. Consider adding calming essential oils such as lavender to enhance the soothing experience.

7. Journaling:

Take a few moments to jot down your thoughts or express gratitude in a journal. This practice helps declutter the mind, allowing you to release any worries or anxieties before bedtime. Reflecting on positive aspects of your day can contribute to a more optimistic mindset.

8. Herbal Tea Ritual:

Sip on a cup of caffeine-free herbal tea, such as chamomile or valerian root, as part of your bedtime routine. Warm and soothing, herbal teas have relaxing properties that can contribute to a peaceful transition into sleep.

9. Progressive Muscle Relaxation (PMR):

Incorporate progressive muscle relaxation into your routine to release physical tension. Starting from your toes and working your way up to your head, consciously tense and then relax each muscle group, promoting a deep sense of relaxation.

10. Limit Stimulants and Heavy Meals:

Avoid stimulants like caffeine and nicotine in the evening, as they can interfere with sleep. Similarly, limit heavy meals close to bedtime to prevent discomfort and indigestion that may disrupt your sleep.

Conclusion: Embracing Tranquility for Restful Nights

Crafting a relaxing bedtime routine is a personal journey of self-care and intentionality. By incorporating these practices into your evening ritual, you create a sacred space for relaxation, allowing the stresses of the day to melt away. Embrace the art of cultivating tranquility in the evenings, and you'll find yourself not only falling asleep more easily but also awakening each morning feeling refreshed and ready to embrace a new day.

CHAPTER FOUR

MENTAL WELLNESS

Mental wellness is a dynamic and fluid state characterized by emotional resilience, cognitive flexibility, and a positive outlook on life. It goes beyond the absence of mental health disorders, embracing a proactive approach to mental health that involves intentional self-care, coping mechanisms, and the cultivation of a supportive and nurturing environment.

Cultivating positive mindset

In the symphony of life, the mindset we choose to adopt serves as a powerful conductor, shaping our experiences, perceptions, and responses to the world around us. Cultivating a positive mindset is not merely an exercise in wishful thinking; it is an intentional and transformative practice that empowers individuals to approach life with optimism, resilience, and a greater capacity for joy. This comprehensive guide explores the art of nurturing a positive mindset, offering practical insights and actionable strategies for those seeking to infuse their lives with a sunnier perspective.

Understanding a Positive Mindset:

A positive mindset is a mental attitude that embraces optimism, hope, and a constructive outlook on life. It involves consciously choosing to focus on the good, seek opportunities for growth, and approach challenges as learning experiences rather than insurmountable obstacles. Cultivating a positive mindset is a journey of self-discovery, self-compassion, and intentional thought patterns.

The Power of Positive Thinking:

Framing Challenges as Opportunities:

A positive mindset reframes challenges as opportunities for growth. Rather than viewing setbacks as failures, individuals with a positive mindset see them as chances to learn, adapt, and emerge stronger.

Gratitude as a Daily Practice:

Practicing gratitude involves acknowledging and appreciating the positive aspects of life. Regularly reflecting on what one is thankful for fosters a mindset focused on abundance rather than scarcity.

Optimistic Self-Talk:
The language we use internally influences our mindset. Cultivating a positive mindset involves practicing optimistic self-talk, replacing self-critical thoughts with affirming and encouraging statements.

Embracing Failure as a Stepping Stone:
Rather than fearing failure, a positive mindset sees it as a natural part of the journey toward success. Each failure becomes a stepping stone, providing valuable lessons and insights.

Celebrating Small Wins:
Acknowledging and celebrating small victories, no matter how minor, contributes to a positive mindset. It reinforces a sense of accomplishment and fuels motivation for future endeavors.

Practical Strategies for Cultivating a Positive Mindset:

Mindfulness and Present Moment Awareness:
Engaging in mindfulness practices, such as meditation and mindful breathing, helps anchor the mind in the present moment. This reduces dwelling on past regrets or worrying about an uncertain future, fostering a positive mindset.

Surrounding Yourself with Positivity:

The company we keep significantly influences our mindset. Surround yourself with positive influences, whether it's supportive friends, inspirational literature, or uplifting media, to create an environment conducive to positive thinking.

Visualizing Success:

Visualization involves mentally picturing successful outcomes and positive scenarios. By visualizing success, individuals can create a mental blueprint for achieving their goals and reinforcing a positive mindset.

Acts of Kindness and Generosity:
Engaging in acts of kindness and generosity not only benefits others but also enhances one's own sense of well-being. Acts of kindness release feel-good hormones, contributing to a positive mindset.

Regular Exercise and Physical Well-Being:
Physical activity has a direct impact on mental well-being. Regular exercise releases endorphins, the body's natural mood enhancers, promoting a positive mindset and reducing stress.

Learning and Growth Mindset:
Cultivating a positive mindset involves adopting a growth mindset. Embrace challenges as opportunities to learn and grow, and view effort as a path to mastery rather than a futile endeavor.

Overcoming Challenges in Cultivating a Positive Mindset:
- Awareness and Mindful Reflection:

Becoming aware of negative thought patterns is the first step in overcoming them. Mindful reflection allows individuals to recognize and challenge negative thoughts, replacing them with more positive alternatives.

- Building Resilience:

Developing resilience involves bouncing back from adversity. Cultivating a positive mindset contributes to resilience by fostering a belief in one's ability to navigate challenges and overcome adversity.

- Seeking Support and Connection:

Positive mindsets thrive in a supportive and connected environment. Seek support from friends, family, or mental health professionals when faced with challenges, fostering resilience and maintaining a positive outlook.

- Conclusion: Radiating Positivity in Every Step

Cultivating a positive mindset is not a destination but a journey, a continuous process of self-discovery and intentional thought patterns. By embracing optimism, gratitude, and a growth mindset, individuals can radiate positivity in every aspect of their lives. As we embark on this journey, we not only enhance our own well-being but also contribute to a more uplifting and compassionate world.

Practices For Mindful Living

In the bustling tapestry of modern life, characterized by constant connectivity and a myriad of responsibilities, the practice of mindful living emerges as a transformative approach to navigating the complexities of the present moment. Mindful living involves intentional awareness, non-judgmental observation, and a commitment to being fully present in each experience. This comprehensive guide explores the practices that form the foundation of mindful living, offering insights and actionable steps for those seeking to infuse their daily lives with greater clarity, presence, and serenity.

Understanding Mindful Living

At its core, mindful living is about embracing the richness of each moment without being entangled in past regrets or future worries. It involves cultivating a heightened awareness of thoughts, emotions, and sensations while fostering a non-reactive and compassionate response to the world around us. Mindful living is not a destination but a continuous journey, an ongoing practice that unfolds in every breath, step, and interaction.

Key Practices for Mindful Living:

- Mindful Breathing:

The breath serves as an anchor to the present moment. Mindful breathing involves paying attention to each inhale and exhale, allowing the breath to guide awareness back to the present when the mind wanders.

- Body Scan Meditation:

The body scan is a practice where attention is systematically brought to each part of the body.

This practice enhances body awareness, releases tension, and fosters a deeper connection between the mind and body.

- **Mindful Eating:**

Mindful eating involves savoring each bite with full attention. It includes appreciating the flavors, textures, and aromas of the food, cultivating a deeper connection to the act of nourishing the body.

- **Walking Meditation:**

Transforming each step into a mindful experience, walking meditation encourages individuals to bring awareness to the sensations of walking. This practice can be done indoors or outdoors, fostering a sense of groundedness.

- **Mindful Observation:**

Engage in mindful observation by paying attention to the details of your surroundings. Whether it's the colors of nature, the sounds in your environment, or the sensations of touch, this practice heightens awareness and presence.

- Mindful Listening:

Actively listen to others with full attention, setting aside judgments and preconceived notions. Mindful listening involves being fully present in conversations, fostering deeper connections and understanding.

- Mindful Work:

Infuse mindfulness into your work routine by bringing full attention to each task. Whether it's typing an email, attending a meeting, or completing a project, approach each task with intentionality and focus.

- Mindful Digital Engagement:

In the age of constant digital connectivity, mindful living extends to our online interactions. Practice mindful scrolling, set boundaries for screen time, and be intentional about the content you consume.

- Mindful Self-Compassion:

Cultivate a kind and compassionate relationship with yourself. When faced with challenges or setbacks, practice self-compassion by acknowledging your feelings without judgment and offering yourself the same kindness you would to a friend.

Overcoming Challenges in Mindful Living:

1. Cultivating Patience:

Mindful living requires patience, especially in the face of a busy or distracted mind. Approach the practice with a gentle and patient attitude, understanding that mindfulness is a skill that develops over time.

2. Managing Expectations:

Release the need for immediate results and perfection. Mindful living is about the journey rather than the destination. Manage expectations and appreciate the small, incremental shifts in awareness.

3. Returning to the Present:

The mind often wanders, and that's perfectly normal. When distractions arise, gently guide your focus back to the present moment. This process of returning to the now is an integral part of mindful living.

Conclusion: A Journey of Self-Discovery and Presence

Mindful living is not a rigid set of rules but a flexible and adaptable approach to experiencing life with heightened awareness. By integrating these practices into daily life, individuals can embark on a journey of self-discovery, presence, and serenity. As we cultivate mindfulness, we not only enhance our own well-being but also contribute to a more mindful and compassionate world.

CHAPTER FIVE

HOLISTIC APPROACHES TO SELF CARE
In the fast-paced rhythm of modern life, the concept of self-care has transcended mere indulgence and transformed into a holistic approach that addresses the intricate interplay of mind, body, and spirit. Holistic self-care is an intentional and comprehensive practice that recognizes the interconnectedness of various facets of well-being. This article explores the principles and practices of holistic self-care, offering insights and actionable steps for those seeking to nurture a sense of balance, vitality, and fulfillment in their lives.

Understanding Holistic Self-Care:

Holistic self-care goes beyond surface-level pampering and encompasses a deeper understanding of the interconnected nature of our well-being. It recognizes that mental, physical, and spiritual health are intertwined and that caring for one aspect inevitably impacts the others. Holistic self-care is not a one-size-fits-all approach; rather, it is a personalized journey of self-discovery and intentional choices that promote overall well-being.

Key Components of Holistic Self-Care:

1. Mindful Practices:

Holistic self-care begins with cultivating mindfulness. Engaging in practices such as meditation, mindful breathing, and present-moment awareness fosters a deep connection with the mind, promoting mental clarity and emotional well-being.

2. Nutrition and Physical Well-Being:

Nourishing the body with a balanced and wholesome diet is a fundamental aspect of holistic self-care. Regular exercise, sufficient sleep, and hydration contribute to physical vitality, energy, and resilience.

3. Emotional Well-Being:

Holistic self-care involves acknowledging and addressing emotional well-being. This includes fostering healthy relationships, setting boundaries, and practicing self-compassion. Emotional well-being contributes significantly to overall life satisfaction.

4. Spiritual Connection:

Regardless of individual beliefs, cultivating a sense of spiritual connection is integral to holistic self-care. This may involve engaging in practices that align with personal spiritual beliefs, such as meditation, prayer, or spending time in nature.

5. Creativity and Expression:

Embracing creativity and self-expression is a powerful component of holistic self-care. Engage in activities that allow for creative expression, whether it's through art, writing, music, or any form of personal expression.

6. Social Connection:

Human connection is a vital element of holistic self-care. Foster meaningful relationships, engage in social activities, and create a supportive network that contributes to emotional and social well-being.

7. Environmental Awareness:
Consideration for the environment is an often-overlooked aspect of holistic self-care. Making eco-friendly choices in daily life, spending time in nature, and fostering a connection with the environment contribute to overall well-being.

Holistic Self-Care Practices:
- Daily Rituals:

Establish daily rituals that promote balance and mindfulness. This may include a morning routine, moments of reflection throughout the day, and calming rituals before bedtime.

- Mindful Movement:

Engage in mindful movement practices such as yoga, tai chi, or qigong. These activities not only contribute to physical well-being but also enhance mental clarity and spiritual connection.

- Holistic Therapies:

Explore holistic therapies that address the mind-body-spirit connection. This may include acupuncture, massage, aromatherapy, or other alternative modalities that promote overall well-being.

- Digital Detox:

Recognize the impact of constant digital connectivity on well-being. Incorporate digital detox periods into your routine, allowing for moments of unplugged and mindful living.

- Educational Pursuits:

Nourish the mind through ongoing education and self-discovery. Engage in learning activities that align with personal interests, fostering a sense of curiosity and intellectual well-being.

Challenges and Strategies in Holistic Self-Care:

1. Time Management:
Prioritize self-care by managing time effectively. Schedule dedicated moments for self-care practices, and view them as non-negotiable appointments with yourself.

2. Balancing Priorities:
Striking a balance between various aspects of well-being can be challenging. Regular self-assessment and reflection help individuals identify areas that may need more attention, ensuring a holistic approach.

3 Overcoming Guilt:
Some individuals may experience guilt or resistance to prioritizing self-care. Recognize that self-care is not selfish; it is an essential investment in overall well-being that enables individuals to show up fully for themselves and others.

Self - Care Rituals for Physical and mental well-being

In the whirlwind of modern life, where demands seem ceaseless and the pace relentless, self-care becomes an imperative practice to sustain balance and well-being. The synergy of physical and mental health forms the cornerstone of overall wellness. This article delves into self-care rituals that intertwine the nurturing of the body and mind, offering practical insights to cultivate a harmonious and resilient sense of well-being.

The Interconnectedness of Physical and Mental Well-Being:

Understanding the intimate connection between physical and mental health is pivotal in crafting effective self-care rituals. The body and mind operate as a symbiotic duo, influencing each other in a continuous dance. Nourishing one aspect inevitably enhances the other, creating a holistic tapestry of well-being.

Self-Care Rituals for Physical Well-Being:
Regular Exercise:

Physical activity is a cornerstone of self-care for the body. Whether it's a brisk walk, a yoga session, or a full workout, regular exercise boosts mood, improves cardiovascular health, and enhances overall physical well-being.

Balanced Nutrition:
Nourishing the body with a well-balanced diet rich in nutrients is a fundamental self-care ritual. Ensure a variety of fruits, vegetables, whole grains, and lean proteins to provide the body with the energy and nutrients it needs.

Adequate Sleep:
Quality sleep is a linchpin for both physical and mental health. Establishing a consistent sleep routine, creating a conducive sleep environment, and prioritizing adequate rest contribute to overall well-being.

Hydration:
Staying well-hydrated is a simple yet powerful self-care practice. Water is essential for bodily functions, and maintaining proper hydration

levels supports physical vitality and cognitive function.

Relaxation Techniques:

Incorporate relaxation techniques into your routine to alleviate physical tension. This may include practices such as deep breathing, progressive muscle relaxation, or a warm bath to soothe muscles and promote relaxation.

Self-Care Rituals for Mental Well-Being:

- Mindfulness Meditation:

Mindfulness meditation is a potent self-care ritual for mental well-being. It involves cultivating present-moment awareness, reducing stress, and promoting a calm and centered state of mind.

- Journaling:

Expressive writing through journaling can be a cathartic self-care practice. Write down thoughts, feelings, and reflections to gain insights into your emotions and foster mental clarity.

- Digital Detox:

Unplugging from digital devices, even for short periods, is a vital self-care ritual for mental well-being. Limit screen time, especially before bedtime, to reduce the impact of digital stimuli on sleep and cognitive function.

- Mindful Breathing Exercises:

Incorporate mindful breathing exercises into your daily routine. Focused breathing techniques, such as diaphragmatic breathing or box breathing, can promote relaxation and reduce the physiological effects of stress.

- Cultivate Gratitude:

Practicing gratitude is a transformative self-care ritual for mental well-being. Regularly reflect on and express gratitude for positive aspects of your life, fostering a positive mindset and emotional resilience.

Integrated Self-Care Rituals:
1. Mindful Movement Practices:

Activities like yoga or tai chi seamlessly integrate physical and mental well-being. These mindful movement practices not only enhance flexibility and strength but also cultivate a focused and tranquil state of mind.

2. Nature Connection:
Spending time in nature is a holistic self-care ritual. Whether it's a walk in the park, a hike, or simply sitting in a garden, nature connection rejuvenates the body and provides a mental sanctuary.

3. Social Connection:
Cultivate meaningful relationships for both physical and mental well-being. Social connection provides emotional support, reduces feelings of isolation, and contributes to overall life satisfaction

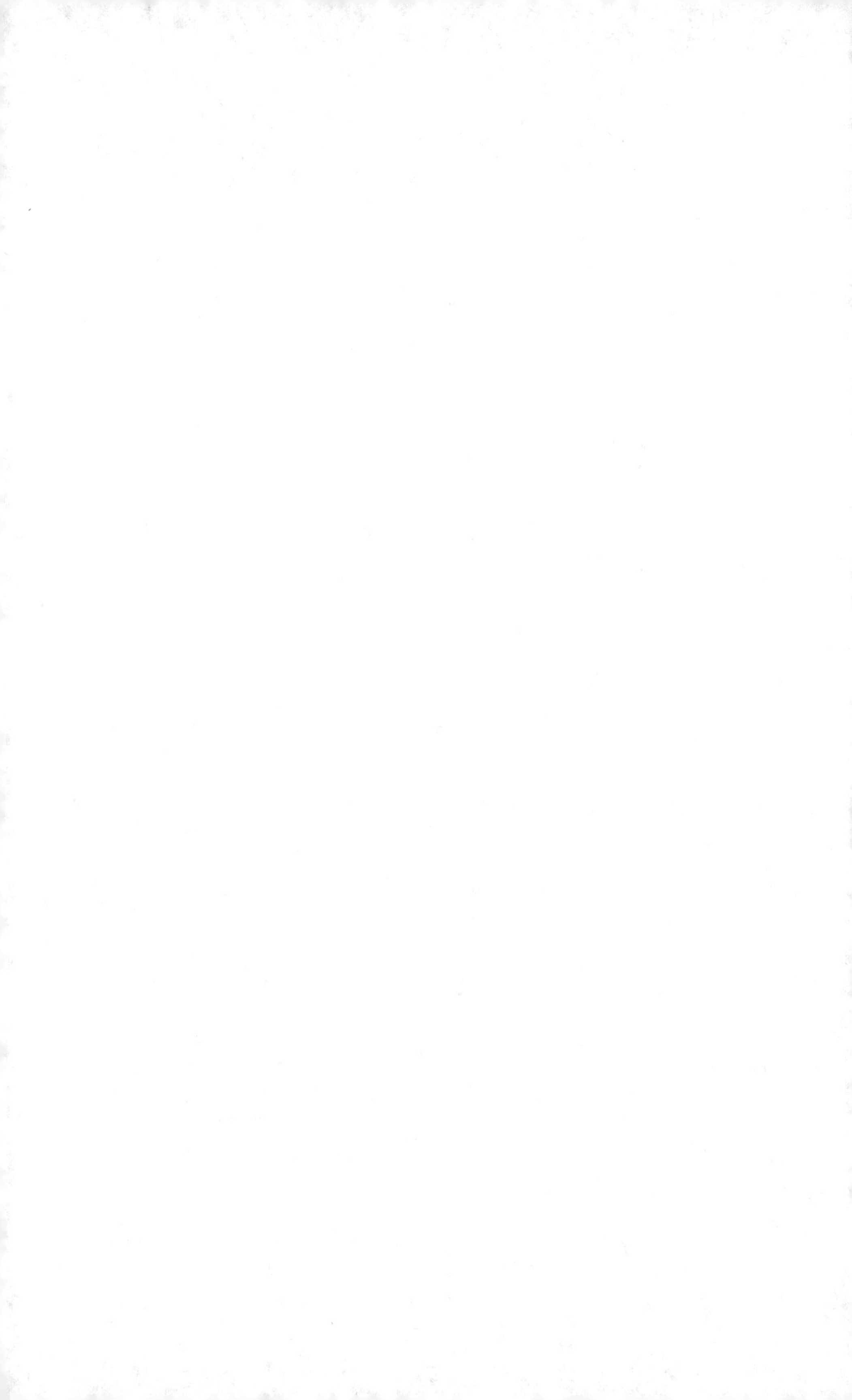